WIPE OUT KIDNEY DISEASES

A GUIDE TO BETTER KIDNEY HEALTH

Copyright@2023

Jerald Lora

TABLE OF CONTENT

CHAPTER ONE

WIPE OUT KIDNEY DISEASES

Kidney is an osmoregulatory organ, a pair of kidney is present in our body which filters blood before sending it back to heart and both kidneys receive 20% blood supply with each cardiac beat. One of the most familiar functions of kidney is urine formation. The kidneys are two large organs placed at the base of the rig cage. There's really one kidney on every side of the spinal cord. It is a major endocrine organ which secretes variety of hormones.

1. RENIN: leads to the production of potent pressor

hormone angiotensin and produces all the following hormones and humoral factors acts.

2. KALLIKRENS: acts on blood protein to produce a vasorelaxing peptide bradykinin.

3. ERTHROPOIETIN: essential for red blood cell formation by bone marrow.

4. 1,25 $CHOHJ_2$ Vitamin D3: essential for calcium homeostasis.

FUNCTIONS

Kidneys are necessary for a healthy body. They are primarily responsible for filtering blood for waste materials, excess water, and other contaminants. The bladder stores these poisons, which are eventually eliminated during urine. Additionally, the kidneys manage the body's pH, sodium, and potassium levels. They generate hormones that control the formation of red blood cells and regulate blood pressure. The kidney also activates a type of vitamin D that aids in calcium absorption. Kidney disease develops when the kidneys become damaged and unable to function properly. Diabetes, high blood pressure, and other chronic conditions may cause harm (long term condition). Kidney illnesses can cause further health issues, including brittle bones, nerve damage, and starvation. If the condition progresses, your kidneys may quit functioning entirely. This indicates that dialysis will be necessary to perform renal functions. Dialysis is a treatment that uses a machine to filter and purify the blood. Although it cannot cure renal illness, it can extend your life.

KIDNEY DISEASE SYMPTOMS

Kidney illness is often undiagnosed until the signs are severe. These symptoms are early indicators that you may be developing renal disease:

• Fatigue
• Difficulty concentrating
• Trouble sleeping
• Poor appetite

• Cramps in the muscles • Swollen feet/ankles

• Morning dry, scaly skin around the eyes

• Frequent urinating, especially at night

Severe signs to indicate progression of renal disease to kidney failure:

• Nausea

• Vomiting

• Loss of Appetite

• Alterations in Urine Output

• Fluid Retention

• Anemia (a decrease in red blood cells)

• Decreased libido

• Sudden increase in potassium levels (hyperkalemia)

• Pericardial inflammation (fluid filled sac that covers the hearts)

Important items to avoid for kidney disease prevention:

1. A terrible decision is to hold urine in the bladder for an inordinate amount of time. A full bladder could cause bladder damage. Urine that lingers in the bladder causes damage to the bladder and promotes the rapid development of bacteria. The disease known as venous insufficiency occurs when urine backs up into the ureter and kidneys. Toxic chemicals can cause kidney infections, followed by urinary tract infections, nephritis, and possibly uremia.

2. Consuming excessive salt: You should consume no more than 5.8 grams of salt per day.

3. Consuming an excessive amount of protein is detrimental to the kidneys. Ammonia, a toxin produced by protein breakdown, is extremely damaging to the kidneys. More meats equal more renal damage.

4. Consuming excessive amounts of caffeine: Caffeine is a common ingredient in sodas and soft drinks. It rises your blood pressure and damages your kidneys. Therefore, you should reduce the amount of coke you consume every day.

5. Not drinking water: Our kidneys must be well hydrated in order to conduct their duties effectively. If we do not consume enough water, toxins can begin to accumulate in the blood because there is insufficient fluid to flush them via the kidneys. Consume more than 10 glasses of water every day. Examine the color of your urine to see if you are drinking enough water; the lighter the hue, the better.

6. Treat all your health issues before it's too late (diabetes, high blood pressure etc.). Regularly assess your health and care for yourself properly.

CHAPTER TWO

DIFFERENT KIDNEY DISEASES

1. ANURIA

Auria, also known as anuresis, occurs when the kidney ceases to produce urine. Typically, the condition is caused by renal illness or injury. Normal 24-hour urine output ranges from 1,000 to 2,000 ml; however, if the urine output is less than 400 ml/24h or less than 12 ml/h in adults, further evaluation is required. It is known as oliguria, whereas auria is characterized by a urine production of less than 100 ml per 24 hours or 1 ml per hour, and by a significant volume of pee (at least 3000ml over 24h). It is known as polyuria.

CAUSES OF AURIA

1. Low blood pressure may be the result of substantial blood loss, severe dehydration from vomiting or diarrhea, or a severe infection that reduces blood flow to the kidneys, resulting in acute renal damage and anuria.

2. **Diabetes:** uncontrolled diabetes can induce metabolic alkalosis. This is one of the acute renal failure reasons that may result in anuria.

3. End-stage renal disease or chronic kidney problems

During this stage, the kidney has lost nearly all of its functions and cannot produce urine.

4. **Kidney stone:** Kidney stones are mineral deposits that resemble stones and are generated when concentrated urine crystallizes the mineral into a solid form. When large enough, these stones can obstruct the entire urinary tract.

5. **Kidney tumors:** Tumors impede kidney function, clog the urethra at multiple levels, and therefore can decrease urinary output.

SIGNS AND SYMPTOMS OF AURIA

1. foot and ankle edema
2. Suffering, discomfort or struggle initiating urination.
3. Hematuria or blood in urine
4. General weakness, reduced hunger and frequent vomiting
5. Fluid retention
6. Recent trouble urinating
7. Decreased visit to the bathroom
8. Blood in your urine
9. Fatigue
10. Intestinal or side pain.

LIFESTYLE REMEDIES TO AURIA

1. Reduce foods with high sugar and fat content
2. More intake of fruit and vegetables as per dietician advice
3. Include low fats products
4. low intake of salt and fat diet
5. Liquefied eating as advised by the doctor
6. Steady somatic activity for at least 30 – 45 minutes a day. Could be walking, cycling and light weight.

2. LONG-LASTING RENAL FAILURE

Chronic renal failure is the gradual deterioration of the kidney's ability to eliminate toxins, concentrate urine, and conserve electrolytes. Chronic kidney failure (CKD), also known as chronic renal disease, is a gradual decline in renal function over months or years. The symptoms of deteriorating kidney function are non-specific and may include general malaise and a diminished appetite. Frequently, chronic kidney disease is discovered through screening of individuals who are known to be at risk for renal problems, such as those with high blood pressure, diabetes, or a blood relative who has chronic kidney disease. Chronic kidney disease may also be diagnosed when it causes one of its known consequences, such as cardiovascular disease, anemia, or pericarditis. A blood test for creatinine can diagnose chronic renal disease. Higher levels of creatinine indicate a feeling glomerular filtration rate (rate at which the kidneys filter blood) and as a result a decrease capability of the kidneys to excrete waste products. Creatinine level may be normal in the early stages of CKD, and the condition is discovered if urinalysis (testing of a urine sample) shows that the kidney is allowing the loss of protein or red blood cells into the urine. To fully investigate the underlying cause of kidney damage various forms of medical making blood tests and often renal biopsy (removing a small sample of kidney tissue) are employed to find out if there is a reversible cause the kidney malfunction.

BASES OF CHRONIC RENAL FAILURE (CKD)

The primary causes of chronic kidney disease are diabetes, nephropathy, hypertension, and glomerulonephritis. Certain geographical regions have a high prevalence of HIV nephropathy, which accounts for nearly 75% of all adult cases. Historically, kidney disease has been categorized according to the renal anatomy implicated as follows:

1. Vascular: comprises major vessel disease, like bilateral renal artery stenosis, and small vessel disease, like ischemic nephropathy, hemolytic – uremic syndrome, and vasculitis.

2. Glomerular: a heterogeneous group subdivided as follows:

• Primary Glomerular disease, including focal segmental glomerulosclerosis and nephritis.

• Secondary Glomerular disease, including diabetic nephropathy and lupus nephritis. Tubulointerstitial, which includes polycystic kidney disease, drug and toxin induce chronic, nephritis and reflux nephropathy obstructive, such as with bilateral kidney stones and prostate enlargement.

CLINICAL SIGNS OF CHRONIC RENEAL FAILURE

Initial signs and symptoms may include:

• Tiredness

• Frequent hiccups

• General sickness feeling

• Headache

• Biliousness vomiting

• Unintended weight loss

• Generalized itching (pruritus)

• Anorexia

• Polyuria

• Nocturia

• Facial enlargement

Later signs and symptoms may include:

• Blood in the vomit or feces, diminished alertness including drowsiness, confusion, delirium, and coma.

• Sensation loss in the hands, feet, or other areas.

• Susceptibility to bruising or bleeding

• Alterations in urine output

• Convulsions or twitching of the muscles

• White crystals are present on and in the skin (uremic frost)

• Hallucinations

• fots

• stupor

Other signs that may be related with this disease:

- Irregular dark or light skin
- Agitation
- Breath odor
- Extreme night time urination
- Extreme thirst
- High blood pressure
- Loss of appetite
- Mail abnormalities
- Paleness
- Diarrhea
- Oliguria
- Dyspnea
- Pain in the chest
- Hiccups

- Cramps
- Bone pains
- Bruises
- Epistaxis
- Complications
- Anemia
- Cardiac temponede
- Changes in blood sugar
- Metabolism
- Congestion heart failure
- Decrease function of whole
- Blood cells
- Decrease immune response
- Decrease libido, impotence
- Dementia

Ionic abnormalities, such as:

- Hyperkalemia signs

- Encephalopathy
- Renal insufficiency
- Breakages
- Outpouring
- High blood pressure
- Increased infections
- Joint disorders
- Liver swelling chapattis
- B or hepatitis C
- Liver failure
- Loss of blood from the digestive track
- Menstrual abnormalities
- Miscarriage and infertility
- Nerve damage
- Pericarditis
- Peripheral neuropathy

- Platelet dysfunction
- Ulcers
- Seizures
- Skin dryness, itching
- Scratching with resultant
- Skin infection
- Weakening of the bones
- Uremic come
- Cardiac arrhymia

GENERAL MANAGEMENT

1. Fluid restriction according to urinary output.
2. Maintain ionic balance
3. Systolic
4. Correction of anemia
5. Protein restriction to 0.5m/kg body weight

6. At advance stage, medical doctors can refer the patient for dialysis or kidney transplantation.

3. NEPHRITIS

Nephritis is the general term used to describe inflammation of the glomerulus, tubules on interstitial tissues in the kidneys. Also, Nephritis is a kind of disease that causes inflammation in the kidney bladder. It generally affects the Interstitial tissues which surround the tubules and the glomerulus present in the kidney.

SIGNS OF NEPHRITIS

1. Hematuria (blood in urine may lead to discoloration of the urine.)

2. Proteinuria or albuminuria (protein in urine may lead to frothy urine.)

3. Edema (Swelling of the face, hand and legs.)

4. Hypertension

5. Hypercholesteremic

6. Lack of kidney function

CAUSES OF NEPHRITIS

Nephritis is frequently caused by infections and poisons, but the most prevalent cause is autoimmunity affecting key organs such as the kidneys.

1. Pyelonephritis: Cellulitis is an illness of the kidney's glomerulus caused by a urinary tract infection.

2. Lupus is an autoimmune disease; lupus nephritis is inflammation of the kidney induced by systemic lupus erythematous (SLE), an autoimmune disease.

3. Athletic nephritis is a form of nephritis caused by intense exercise.

TYPES OF NEPHRITIS

1. **Glomerulonephritis:** it involves damage to the filters in the kidney.

2. Intercellular nephropathy damages the area between the kidney and liver glomerulus and is usually accompanied by irritation of the capillaries or longer durations nephritis.

THINGS YOU DO THAT ARE KILLING YOUR KIDNEY

1. Don't empty your bladder when you're pressed

2. Eating excess salt:

Consuming too much salt on a regular is bad for your health. Our kidneys break down 95% of sodium from the food we eat. This means that high salt intake makes the kidney to work harder just to remove the salt. This can in turn lead to poor kidney functioning and increased water retention.

3. Lack of excess water everyday

Due to the fact that your kidneys, like the rest of your body, require adequate water, dehydration might reduce the blood flow to your kidneys. If there is less blood flow, your blood becomes thicker, hampering your body's capacity to eliminate toxins. Obviously, you are aware that passing urine is a method for removing toxins from the body, and that sufficient water is required for this. Another advantage of drinking a lot of water is that it accelerates weight loss. Individuals on a diet must take note.

4. Excessive protein consumption is detrimental. Consuming excessive protein can raise the chance of developing renal disease.

5. You take painkiller always:

Sadly, painkillers and analgesics are harmful to the kidneys, despite the fact that some individuals make it a practice to take them to reduce swelling and fever.

6. Many individuals are guilty of consuming too much sugar, correct? In addition to salt, sugar is also a kidney foe because it can contribute to diminished renal function. Avoid sugary beverages to maintain healthy kidneys.

7. Smoking

The national agency advises that smoking is detrimental to our health. Smoking is hazardous to your health, including your kidneys. The fact that smoking can promote hypertension is one factor.

8. Abusive drunk

If you consume excessive alcohol, you will eventually destroy your kidneys and impair your health. Knowing that certain individuals would come up with something that must kill a man. You are correct, but would you rather hasten your demise by ignorance? I just believe moderation is vital.

PRECAUTION ON KIDNEY DISEASE

1. Prolonging the usage of toilet:
Urine should not be stored in the bladder for an extended period of time. The kidney excretes between

one and three liters of pee daily; a full bladder can be harmful. Urine that remains in the bladder multiplies bacteria rapidly. Once the pee has refluxed (returned) to the urethra, it flows to the pelvic cavity and kidney. According to the poisonous material's capacity to generate refluxed action and activation, the kidney may lose its capability to keep metabolic homeostasis, resulting in a dramatic shift in fluid, electrolyte, and acid-base balance. They cause nephritis and even uremia by infecting the urinary tract and the nephrons that filter the volume of urine in the kidney.

2. Consuming excessive salt:

Salt intake should not exceed 5.8 grams daily. After cooking, you should not add additional salt to the food.

3. Our kidneys require a precise amount of water in order to operate properly; therefore, we must dehydrate them adequately in order for them to work properly. If you don't drink enough water, your kidneys won't be able to eliminate toxins from the body, leading to heart failure, kidney failure, etc. Yet, we should strive to consume a certain amount of water:

- Upon awakening in the morning, have two glasses of water.
- Before taking a bath, have two glasses of water.
- Have one glass of water 20 minutes prior to a meal.
- Have 2 glasses of water half an hour after a meal.
- Consume 1 glass of water before going to bed at least 8 liters of water.

4. Limit soda consumption:
consuming too much soda raises blood pressure, which in turn causes

renal dysfunction. This causes the kidney to suffer by strangulating the kidney's neck. So, you should reduce your daily intake of cake and soda.

5. Minimize red meat consumption

6. Avoid sodium consumption if you have been diagnosed with renal disease. If you're diagnosed with renal failure, you should consume a high amount of carbohydrates and a low amount of protein and potassium.

7. Those diagnosed with renal illness should weigh themselves daily and report any gram fluctuations or weight loss.

CHAPTER THREE

HOW TO IDENTIFY KIDNEY FAILURE?

1. Dull bilateral, frank pain and abdomen tenderness
2. Fever
3. Chills
4. Nausea
5. Vomiting
6. Frequency ad urgency of urination
7. Dysuria (excessive increase test)
8. Foul (smelling urine)
9. Obvious distress
10. Lethargy
11. Anorexic

12. Crackles or elevated blood pressure

13. Headache

14. Pallor

15. Dry and discolored skin

KIDNEY STONES:

Renal (ithrasis, Nephrothrasis) are mineral and sodium deposits that form in the kidneys. Kidney stones can damage any part of the urinary tract, from either the kidneys to the bladder, due to their multiple sources. Typically, pebbles form when urine gets overly concentrated, enabling minerals to solidify and agglomerate. Kidney stones can be super traumatic to pass, but if diagnosed and treated promptly, they normally do not result in permanent damage. Depending on the conditions, you may just require pain medicine and substantial quantities of water to remove a kidney stone. In certain instances, such as when stones become lodged in the urinary tract, are accompanied by a urinary tract infection, or cause complications, surgery may be necessary. If you are at a high risk of developing recurrent kidney stones again, your physician may recommend prophylactic measures to reduce your risk.

SYMPTOMS OF KIDNEY STONE

A kidney stone might not even create problems till it shifts inside the kidney or enters the ureter, the tube that connects the kidney to the urine. At this point, you may feel the following signs and symptoms. Extreme pain in the side and back, just below the ribs, radiating to the lower abdomen and groin. Pain that arrives in waves and varies in intensity.

Urinary Discomfort:

Urine that is pink, red, or brown, murky, and has a bad odor. Nausea and vomiting, a continuous need to urinate, and an increase in urination frequency.

41

Symptoms of an infection include fever and chills, along with infrequent urination. As a kidney stone passes through the urinary tract, the pain it causes may shift or intensify. Commonly, there is no specific cause for kidney stones, but various risk factors can increase your likelihood of developing them. Kidney stones occur when a person's urine contains more crystal-forming chemicals, such as calcium, oxalate, and uric acid, than the urine's fluid can dilute. In addition, your urine may lack chemicals that prevent crystals from staying together, producing an excellent environment for kidney stone formation.

DIFFERENT KINDS OF KIDNEY STONES

Understanding the forms of kidney stones aids in identifying the reason and may provide hints on how to lower your chances of developing additional kidney stones. Attempt to save your kidney if you lose one so that you can bring it to your doctor for analysis. Among the several types of kidney stones are: -

1. Calcium stones: the majority of kidney stones are calcium stones, typically in the form of calcium oxalate. Oxalate occurs naturally in food and is also produced by the liver on a daily basis. Many fruits and vegetables, as well as nuts and chocolate, contain a significant amount of oxalate. High levels of vitamin D, intestinal bypass surgery, and a number of metabolic disorders can raise the quantity of calcium or oxalate in urine due to dietary variables. Calcium stone can also be composed of calcium phosphate. This form of stone occurs more frequently in metabolic circumstances such as renal tubular acidosis. It may also be linked to migraine headaches or the use of certain seizure drugs, such as topiramate (Topamax).

2. Stones of Sturite: Infections, such as urinary tract infections, lead to the development of struvite stones. Without many symptoms or warnings, these stones can develop swiftly and become extremely enormous.

3. Uric acid stones: uric acid stones can occur in people who don't drink enough fluids or lose too much fluid, who consume a high-protein diet, or who have gout. Also, certain hereditary characteristics may raise your risk for uric acid stones.

4. Crystine stones: these stones arise in individuals with an inherited disease that causes the kidneys to discharge an excessive amount of a certain amino acid (cystinuria). Family and personal history are among the risk factors that enhance the likelihood of acquiring kidney stones. If a family member has kidney stones, your risk of developing them increases. And if you've had one or more kidney stones before, you're at a greater risk of having another one. Not drinking enough water each day can raise your risk of kidney stones. Individuals who live in warm areas and sweat profusely may be at a greater risk than others.

5. High-protein, high-sodium (salt), and high-sugar diets:

May raise the risk of some forms of kidney stones. This is particularly true for diets heavy in salt. An excessive amount of salt in the diet increases the amount of calcium that the kidneys must filter and considerably raises the chance of developing kidney stones.

6. Obesity, as measured by a high body mass index (BMI), a big waist circumference, and weight gain, is associated with an increased risk of kidney stones.

7. Digestive illnesses and surgery: Inflammatory bowel disease, frequent diarrhea, and weight gain have been associated with an increased risk of kidney stones. Inflammatory bowel disease, or chronic diarrhea can induce alterations in the digestive process that influence calcium and water absorption, hence raising the quantities of stone-forming chemicals in the urine. Additional medical problems that can raise the incidence of kidney stones include renal tubular acidosis, crystimuria, hyperparathyroidism, infections, and certain drugs.

DETOXIFY YOUR KIDNEY AND LIVER

Kidneys are crucial for the function of our body. They assist in the detox process and are crucial in removing our toxins and undesired chemicals from the body. The kidneys maintain the balance and health of our bodies, but they are also susceptible to kidney stones, which form when an excess of mineral deposits in the kidneys. Large kidney stones can cause excruciating pain and even obstruct urine flow.

The liver and the kidney are essential organs of the body. The liver aids in waste elimination and processes numerous nutrients and medications, while the kidneys are responsible for eliminating waste and excess fluid through the urine. The liver and kidneys are extremely important organs that should be cared for properly, as they are susceptible to gradual deterioration that, if left untreated, might result in disease or failure. Periodically, the liver and kidneys must be detoxified in order to eliminate poisonous compounds that can cause illness or death. Detoxification is the physiological or medicinal elimination of harmful chemicals from the body. Detoxification cleansed poisons that the liver and kidneys may not be able to handle, and it gave the organs a much-needed rest. Frequent liver detoxification can greatly increase its function and encourages the breakdown of body fat cells. There are herbs that can be used naturally to cleanse the liver and kidneys in order to prevent disease and failure of these organs. These herbs include qualities that not only purge the body of toxins, but also mend damaged tissues in the kidney and liver until they resume normal function. Following are the names and advantages of the herbs listed below.

1. Sour sop leaves: The leaves of the sour sop plant are considered to be low in calories and high in fiber and vitamin C. It contains a tiny quantity of niacin, riboflavin, folate, and iron. Its leaves, fruits, and stems all contain therapeutic properties. It is rich in antioxidants, which help prevent cell damage and reduce the chance of developing chronic diseases.

2. The vitamin C and iron content of guava leaves is quite high. It helps to strengthen the immune system, consequently minimizing the risk of numerous illnesses. In addition, it contains chemicals in its extracts that may impede the proliferation of cancer cells. It should be mentioned

that those with low blood pressure should not consume guava leaves for more than two weeks, as they drop blood pressure. To eliminate toxins from the body, both soursop and guava leaves can be utilized. Using two leaves is more effective than using one.

PREPARATION

1. Combine five leaves of soursop and five leaves of guava.

2. Rinse them well with purified water

3. Place in a clean pot with 2 cups of clean water.

4. Bring to a boil for five minutes and leave it cool. 5. Sift the mixture and consume warm. Effective dosage is

one-half cup in the morning and at night.

Moreover, consume nutritious foods, avoid junk food, and eat more fruits and vegetables.

HOW TO USE KIDNEY BEANS TO CURE KIDNEY STONES DISEASE?

According to German Physician kidney beans are an exceedingly proficient cure for kidney stones. Extract the seed from the shells before slicing the pods and placing around (60) grams in four liters of boiling water for four hours. The liquid must be strained through fine filters and cooled for approximately eight hours.

The fluid should then be consumed every two hours for the next 24 hours. After then, it may be taken multiple times per week. This medication will not be effective if it has been cooked for more than twenty-four hours.

RENAL STONE REMEDIES

1. Vinegar from apples:

Vinegar from apples is a highly effective treatment for a range of ailments, especially kidney stones. In addition to breaking up and flushing away stones, daily ingestion of around 2 tablespoons of apple cider vinegar can prevent future occurrences. Take an apple cider vinegar tonic first thing in the morning, again around midday, and a third time in the evening to reap the health advantages of this miraculous natural cure and eliminate kidney stones simultaneously. Simply combine 2 teaspoons of raw organic unfiltered ACV with 4 ounces of water and a natural sweetener such as honey or stevia powder.

2. Lemon juice + olive oil

Those with smaller kidney stones can use a mixture of lemon juice and olive oil to help break them up and flush them out. This treatment may not be appropriate for those with larger kidney stones. Combine 1/4 cup each of lemon juice and olive oil, then drink and follow with at least 8 ounces of water. Ensure that you use only high-quality components so that you don't mistakenly introduce something to your body (such as sugar or H.F.C.S) that would exacerbate the disease.

3. Watermelon juice

Water is essential for eliminating kidney stones. It is also rich in potassium, a kind of salt that aids in the dissolution of kidney stones. Watermelon is diuretic and stimulates the production of urine. In addition to consuming as much water as possible, you should consume one to two juices every day.

4. Pomegranate juice

According to a 2008 study, pomegranate juice inhibits the production of certain types of kidney stones. If you suspect that you may be at risk for kidney stones. Eat one or two servings of pomegranates, which are similarly rich in antioxidants.

REMEDIES FOR EDEMA OR WATER RETENSION

Do you regularly feel swollen? Or to have feet that are so swollen that you cannot wear shoes? You are likely impacted by edema, or fluid retention, as it is more often called. This is the result of excessive fluid collection in the tissue. It commonly affects the feet and legs, but can also affect other regions of the body. It can be caused by a high sodium intake (too much salt), poor circulation, lack of exercise, vitamin deficiencies, venous insufficiency (a problem with the blood flow from the legs to the heart), stress, pregnancy-related frustration, warm weather, altitude allergies, high blood pressure, heart problems, kidney problems, chronic lung disease, liver disease, thyroid disorders, certain medications, and oral contraceptives. Typically, water retention produces edema of the affected areas. It can also cause stiffness in the joints, a change in weights, a sense of bloat, higher blood pressure and increasing pulse etc. The following are effective home remedies for water retention:

1. Dandelion

Reduce salt levels to prevent clogging. According to a 2009 study published in the journal of alternative and complementary medicine, dandelion has a diuretic impact. This makes dandelion an excellent remedy for removing excess water from the body. It is also a good source of potassium, which helps lower sodium levels in the body. In addition, its magnesium content makes it perfect for alleviating premenstrual bloating. Infuse a teaspoon of dried dandelion herb in a cup of boiling water for approximately ten minutes. This tea may be filtered and consumed up to three times daily. Like dandelion, parsley has good diuretic qualities; 2 teaspoons of dried parsley leave in one cup of hot water. Let infused for 10 minutes. You can also have a blend of fresh parsley juice and lemon juice three times per day.

2. Epsom salt

To remove poisons and eliminate fluids. A magnesium sulphate (Epsom salt) bath can assist eliminate water retention. It aids in eliminating extra fluids and poisons from the body. The soothing bath also calms aching muscles and nerves. Put two cups of Epsom salt into a hot bath, soak for approximately fifteen minutes, and repeat up to three times each week.

3. Lemon juice

Lemon juice aids in the elimination of extra fluid and pollutants. Combine two tablespoons of lemon juice with one cup of boiling water. You can also use honey to sweeten it.

Use this cure once a day for a few days, or until you see an improvement.

4. Fennel seeds

Fennel seeds stimulate the elimination of salt in the body. According to studies, fennel acts as a diuretic and increases the excretion of salt and water by the kidneys. Moreover, it reduces the buildup of toxins in the body. Improves digestion and reduces gas. Pour a teaspoon of fennel seeds into a cup of warm water, cover, and let soak for 10 minutes. After straining, have this tea three times daily until symptoms improve. Nettle is an excellent natural diuretic for preventing and lowering water retention.

Preparation

Bring 1 cup of water and 1 teaspoon of nettle root extract to a boil. Let this tea too steep for approximately 10 minutes, then consume it three times per day until you see an improvement.

5. Cranberry juice

Cranberry juice is a common home treatment for treating water retention due to its liquid-regulating action in the body and its diuretic qualities. It is also abundant in minerals like magnesium, potassium, and calcium, which aid in maintaining fluid equilibrium. Each day, consume one cup of cranberry juice. In addition, you can take cranberry pills.

6. Apple cider vinegar

Apple cider vinegar alleviates water retention by refilling the body's potassium levels, which aids in regulating salt levels. Mix one teaspoon of apple cider vinegar with one glass of water and consume twice daily. Ten minutes of soaking your feet in a warm foot bath consisting of equal parts apple cider vinegar and hot water will minimize foot odor. Onion contains diuretic and blood purifying properties. It will also prevent kidney stones from forming. Boil some raw onions in four cups of water, add salt to taste, filter the solution, and consume two to three cups every day for several days.

In addition to these therapies, you can try increasing your consumption of diuretic foods including cabbage, cucumber, watercress, celery, bananas, pineapple, and watermelon. Moreover, drink lots of water throughout the day (dehydration causes the body to retain water), restrict your salt consumption, drink less alcohol, and exercise often.

CHAPTER FOUR

KIDNEY TREATMENT

1. CHLOROPHYLL DETOXIFICATION

The chlorophyll for recurrent infections, kidney stones, gallstones, fallopian tube blockage due to infections, and boosting the body's immunity. Consider the following components:

- Chlorophyll powder
- The UTI herbal tea Garlic
- Cinnamon
- Fresh ginger Lemon
- One liter of boiling-hot water Jar

Preparation

Instead of pounding or crushing the garlic, push it to break using two cloves and a knife. Crush 2 to 4 cinnamon sticks and a healthy amount of ginger. Prepare 1 lemon by slicing it. Place the aforementioned components in a jar without squeezing them. Then, add 1 liter of boiling water. Add 1 tablespoon of chlorphy11 powder, add 1 tablespoon of UTI tea and thoroughly combine. Cover the jar's contents and allow them to cool. It should cool without becoming cold. Let it be lukewarm.

Usage

- Reduce the content until only the solution is left.

- Add freshly squeezed lemon juice and honey to the mixture.

- Consume this entire stuff at ounce in the morning.

- Give yourself 30 to 60 minutes before consuming food or liquids. By this time frame, you will have eliminated all poisons via urine and feces.

What to do next:

- Consume apples, watermelon, cucumbers, and oranges that are green.

- Drink half a liter of water alongside
- Eat nothing before noon
- Eat lunch
- Also repeat in the evening what was done in the morning. Wait an hour after consuming the detox solution before consuming watermelon, apples, cucumbers, and oranges.
- Do not consume supper
- Do this cleanse for 10-30 days for optimal results.

2. PAPAYA ROOT FOR TREATMENT OF KIDNEY DISEASE

Papaya is also known as pawpaw and is native to the tropical lowlands of the United States. It is a member of the family fabaceae, and its scientific term is "carica papaya." It is a short-lived plant that can reach a height of 30 feet. The papaya's leaves are orange-red, yellow-green, and orange-yellow, while its pulp is orange-colored. Not only are its fruits nutritious, but the entire plant, including its leaves, stems, and roots, has therapeutic use. The papaya tree roots extract recognized for its anti-urolithiatic action. This action prohibits the deposition of components responsible for kidney stone formation. This, in turn, prevents the formation of urinary stones. Take two equal portions of papaya roots and boil them for 10–15 minutes in two cups of water. Now filter the herbal solution using a tea strainer and consume it regularly.

3. BITTERCOLA AND MALT FOR KIDNEY TREATMENT

I'm certain that by now we have all understood that conventional therapy is just as effective, if not more so, than our modern pharmaceuticals. The benefit or advantage of herbal or traditional medicine over modern medication is that you can make it for free. All you need is to follow instruction correctly. It is safer than white drugs, the majority of which, if not all, have several adverse effects.

The ingredients of an effective treatment for kidney disease are simple and straightforward. You only require three seeds of bitter kola and one bottle of malt. Then, ground the bitter kola, combine it with the malt, and consume everything at once.

This medication is highly helpful for refilling blood (in anemic patients) and bolstering the immune system to combat oncoming illnesses.

Also, it will keep your liver and kidneys in excellent condition.

4. CHANCA PIEDRRA FOR KIDNEY TREATMENT

Lab grade chancea piedra is a plant that has traditionally been used to cure kidney stones. Since 2002, when a study demonstrated chanca piedra's efficacy in the treatment of kidney stones, interest in this rare plant has increased dramatically. Chanca piedra prevents the production of kidney stones. So, ingesting this natural cure can minimize your risk of developing kidney stones greatly. In addition, it facilitates the passage of stone minerals, resulting in pain reduction. According to proponents of Chanca piedra, its ingestion provides practically rapid pain alleviation. Remember to stay hydrated after taking Chanca piedra to aid pass kidney stones. This miracle plant has gone unnoticed for decades. Many individuals are unaware of what the creator has given us. We utilize these items for cooking, but we are unaware of their role beyond garnishing food. You spend hundreds of dollars on medications when the creator gave you a natural "drug" for nothing!

5. PUMPKIN LEAVES

This inexpensive leaf packs a great deal of power. As well as being rich in vitamin A, vitamin C, iron, and calcium, it has numerous other healing benefits. Its vitamin A content aids in the treatment of eye problems. The vitamin C aids in wound healing by promoting the formation of scar tissue to cover the wound. In addition, it helps maintain strong bones, skin, and teeth. This is because pumpkin leaves contain antioxidants and anti-inflammatory qualities. It is employed in the therapy of the illness. It also includes chlorophy11, saponins, tannis, phenolic chemicals, flavonoids, and phytosterols, which allow the leaves to shrink tumors and kill cancer cells. This leaf is excellent for liver and kidney conditions

HOW TO APPLY

Mix enough ingredients in a blender. Using a net sieve, drain the juice after blending. Consume one cup of the juice in the morning and evening.

6. BLACK CARAWAY IS A TREATMENT FOR KIDNEY DISEASES

- Half a teaspoon of black caraway oil
- seven grains of panaceas powder
- one teaspoon of honey
- one cup of water.

PREPARATION

In a cup of warm water, combine half a tea spoon of honey and half a tea spoon of black caraway oil, then dilute the concoction and take it twice daily. This therapy is also effective for chronic cough and also treatment duration is 21days.

7. GLOMERULAR COLIC (KIDNEY PAIN)

Add 250 grains of black fennel and crush them together with one cup of honey. Take two teaspoons of this combination, combine it with a half cup of water and a half teaspoon of black caraway oil, and use it daily. The duration of treatment is up to twenty-one days.

HOW TO DETOXIFY / CLEANSE YOUR KIDNEYS

INGREDIENTS

- Bitter leaf
- Water melon leaf
- Stoke breaker leaf

PREPARATIONS

Crush these leaves and collect the water extracted from them in a secure container. Two table spoons twice every day. Warning: Wait 24 hours for the bitter leaves to subside. Herbs are a solid treatment for kidney disorders; in this context, we will focus on parsley as an herb for kidney cleansing. Parsley naturally cleanses the kidneys of impurities and aids in the elimination of kidney stones. Frequent use of parsley tea maintains a healthy urinary system and normal blood pressure. Typically, as the years pass, our kidneys filter the blood by removing unwanted organisms and individuals. Yet, as time passes, salt builds, necessitating a cleaning process; the question is how we can overcome this.

ACTIONS TO TAKE

1. Wash a bunch of parsley or cilantro (coriander leaves) before using it.

2. Then, chop it into little pieces, place it in a pot, cover it with clean water, and boil it for ten minutes.

3. After ten minutes, allow the mixture to cool, then strain it into a clean bottle and place it in the refrigerator to cool.

4. Consume one glass each day, and you will detect all salt and other collected toxins leaving your kidney through urination, as well as a previously unfelt difference. Parsley

(cilantro) is recognized as the most effective and natural kidney cleanser.

THREAT RELATED WITH OVER WEIGTH

Kidney disease: - the kidneys are responsible for filtering blood and maintaining blood. Nevertheless, when fat accumulates within them and presses on blood vessels, or when the blood arteries that supply them with blood get blocked, it becomes harder for them to perform their function. This condition can cause a harmful accumulation of waste in the body. Obesity can contribute directly to kidney disease, despite the fact that it can also be a consequence of diabetes and high blood pressure. Kidney infections are life-threatening conditions. So, it is essential that you consult a physician and utilize home remedies to alleviate case symptoms or pair. Moreover, home treatments can be utilized to prevent UTIS and enhance kidney function.

CHAPTER FIVE

NATURAL DRINKS TO PREVENT KIDNEY STONES

1. DRINK WITH BASIL

Basil is a plant that helps lower uric acid levels in the body, hence avoiding kidney stone formation. Two basil leaves per day can be chewed or brewed into a tea to aid the expulsion of the stone components.

PREPARATION

- 1 teaspoon of fresh basil leaves
- 1 glass scalding water (250ml)
- Honey

Put the basil leaves to the water that is boiling and let them steep for a few minutes. Eliminate from high temperature and allow to cool. Have one cup of this beverage every morning.

2. DRINK CELERY

Celery is widely used as a condiment, garnish, or side dish for other dishes, and it aids in the elimination of toxins from the body, so preventing their accumulation. Kidney stones aid in the dissolution of existing kidney stones. Due to its diuretic qualities, celery is advised for the treatment of urinary tract illnesses.

INGREDIENTS

- 2 celery ribs
- 3 servings of water (600ml)

PREPARATION

Cleanse and slice the celery stalks.
Combine them with water until a
homogenous solution is obtained.
Consume one glass of this juice daily.

3. DRINK WITH NETTLE LEAF

Being a natural diuretic, this plant
aids in the elimination and prevention
of kidney stones. Nettle tea is an
excellent method for preventing many
infections.

INGREDIENTS

- 2 teaspoons of stinging nettle
  leaves
- 1 ounce of water (250 ml)
- honey versus stevia

PREPARATION

Bring water to a boil, then add nettle leaves. Let the mixture to simmer for 10 minutes over low heat. Drain and chill the liquid. Have this tea twice or three times every day for two weeks, according to your tastes.

4. DRINK WITH RADISH

This plant possesses characteristics that aid in renal cleansing and prevent the formation of kidney stones. To prevent or treat this condition, you can produce radish juice from the roots and leaves.

INGREDIENTS

- 1 radish.
- 1 ounce of water (200ml).
- Honey

PREPARATION

Shave the radish and remove the stem and grate the fruit. Combine shredded radish with water in order to extract its juice. Add some honey and have a glass of this juice before breakfast and dinner, preferably. Get caraway leaves (Ebolo in Yoruba). Boil it and consume the water solution as frequently as possible. You may include honey. Get fresh calotropis proceca (bomubomu leaf) and boil it with water and honey, if desired. Consume it morning and evening.

DOSAGE

Consume one tiny glass cup of it daily. This cup is consumed daily.

This will improve your kidneys and increase urine production.

5. Fresh coconut tree roots and fresh leaves of orange and lime

PREPARATION/ DOSAGE

Begin to boil the fresh coconut tree roots with leaves of orange and lime with water and consume. Two full glasses per day for four weeks.

HEALTH BENEFITS OF SOME DRINKS AND FRUITS

1. ZOBO DRINK

The Zobo beverage is a popular beverage. It is produced from the leaves of the Roselle plant (Hibiscus sabdariffa) and is common with Nigerians. This vibrant crimson beverage is popular for both daily consumption and as a party drink.

This beverage is readily available, inexpensive, pleasant, refreshing, and has numerous health benefits. Because the Roselle leaf has a naturally sweet flavor, most zobo drink enthusiasts and restaurants do not add sugar to their drinks. A handful of them continue to consume low-cholesterol sugar for whatever reason, perhaps because they are so fond of sugar. This unique characteristic is what distinguishes zobo, since it provides a naturally sweet taste that is harmless and poses no health risks. Fortunately, the health benefits of zobo drink are not limited to just one and are, in fact, virtually limitless, since it provides nothing but a natural flavor, organic essence, and uncontaminated, fresh nutrients. Also, you should be aware of the healthy components contained in zobo drink. This solely applies to the roselles leaf and demonstrates that the benefits of adding additional essences to your zobo beverage can vary and increase. Some of these nutrients are antioxidants that are water-soluble. Antibacterial properties, enzyme inhibitors, and a high content of antioxidants.

The nutrients and beneficial essence included in a zobo drink, notably in the Roselle leaf, are effective in preventing and curing diseases such as high blood pressure and constipation, diabetes and constipation. According to a study conducted by the United States Department of Agriculture, zobo drink is very good at curing. Such ailments and health issues include hypertension or high blood pressure, diabetes, and constipation. As previously said, those with kidney problems are encouraged to consume zobo drink since it includes 15 to 30 percent organic acid. This technique increases the kidney's ability to filter out waste products such as urie and oxalic acid. These two wastes can create a kidney stone, which would become extremely weighty as it grows larger.

2. BANANA STEM JUICE - REMEDY FOR KIDNEY STONE

We are all aware of the health advantages of bananas, but many of us miss the benefits of banana stems. The juice taken from the soft interior region of the banana stem includes a variety of nutrients that can aid in the treatment of numerous health conditions. Banana stem juice, which is rich in fiber, vitamin B6, and potassium, is advised for kidney stone dissolution. If you suffer from gall bladder stones, include banana stem in your diet at least once each week.

The combination of banana stem juice and lime juice is an effective treatment for kidney stones. This cure for kidney stones involves soaking a cup of chopped banana stem in water for roughly an hour. Place the banana stem and water in a blender and process until the juice is extracted. Add lemon juice and a bit of salt after straining the liquid. Consume one cup of banana stem juice every day on an empty stomach in the morning to dissolve kidney stones. Moreover, banana stem juice is quite efficient for treating kidney infections.

3. BENEFITS OF ORANGE JUICE WITH HONEY

Orange is one of the most potent fruits God made, a fact that is unknown to the general public. Orange juice can treat over 12 severe diseases, including kidney stones. Kidney stones are tiny mineral deposits that build in the kidneys and frequently produce symptoms such as severe pain, nausea, and blood in the urine. Orange juice can increase the pH of urine, making it more alkaline. It has been discovered that a higher, more alkaline urine pH may benefit in kidney stone prevention.

PREPARATION

Every night, mix a half glass of orange juice with two teaspoons of honey and consume. To strengthen the body.

4. COCONUT ROOTS FOR GALL BLADDER

The roots of the coconut tree can be utilized to treat gallbladder, urinary, and kidney-related disorders.

When cool, consume four or five thoroughly cleansed roots boiled in moderately salted water.

5. BREAD FRUIT LEAVES FOR KIDNEY STONE CURE

Bread fruit leaf, stone breaker leaf, Bitter kola, add some potassium and along with clean water, cook them. Constantly consume it.

6. PAPAYA SEEDS PHYTONUTRIENTS

The effectiveness of papaya seeds in preventing and treating sickness is quite beneficial. The nutrients in papaya seeds assist cure liver cirrhosis and promote kidney health, thereby averting renal failure. It includes the alkaloid caprine, which kills intestinal worms and amoeba parasites. The papain in papaya seeds aids in protein digestion.

7. MANGO LEAVES

We all enjoy eating mangoes, but how many mango leaves are there? There is no doubt that both mango and its leaves have numerous benefits. Nevertheless, how many of us are familiar with diseases that mango leaves may treat? When young and fragile, mango leaves are crimson or purple and grow to a dark green tint with a pale underside. These leaves are vitamin C, B, and A purified. Also, they are abundant in other nutrients. The mango leaves retain potent antioxidant effects due to their high flavonoid and phenol content. Mango leaves include a multitude of medicinal and therapeutic effects. The mango leaves aid in the treatment of renal and gallstones. The daily consumption of a boil mango leaf assists in removing stones and rinsing them. Numerous individuals testified to the efficacy of consuming mango leaf tea or mango leaf powder in dissolving kidney stones, hence alleviating severe discomfort. linked with the passage of big kidney stones Mango leaves are also reported to aid in the dissolution of gallbladder stones.

8. SCENT LEAVES FOR KIDNEY CLEANSES

To cleanse the kidneys, liver, and gallbladder, boil the smell and garden egg leaves. Following one week of the aforementioned herbal tea. Blend small beetroots, ginger, three garlic cloves, one red onion ball, and fresh ginger with water. Three times per day for ninety days.

9. BENEFITS OF TOMATOES

Tomatoes are an extremely versatile ingredient. They are fantastic when eaten fresh, in salads, or on sandwiches, and when cooked, they acquire a delightful sweetness. Due to their strong acid content, they are ideal for canning. Tomatoes are such an integral part of the American diet that it's difficult to think they were previously deemed poisonous. Not until the mid-1800s did they become a staple diet in the United States.

Only one daily serving of tomato-based foods can have a tremendously positive influence on your health. If consumed daily, they have the ability to prevent and treat a dozen ailments, including heart disease. This is an essential fruit to have in your diet. They supply an abundance of natural vitamins and minerals to the body, including vitamin A, vitamin K, vitamin B, B3, B5, B6, B7, vitamin C, folic acid, magnesium, chromium, choline, zinc, and phosphorus. Tomatoes function as a disinfectant to prevent diarrhea and prevent the formation of kidney stones and gall bladder stones over time. They also significantly reduce the increase in symptoms of the lower urinary tract. Tomato juice should be consumed every day in the morning to lower the risk of kidney disorders.

CHAPTER SIX

HOME REMEDY FOR KIDNEY DISEASES

INGREDIENTS

- Lemon leave
- Apple cider vinegar
- Coconut liquid
- Renny beans
- Olive oil
- Scent leaf
- Water melon

PREPARATION

1. 1 litre of citrus juice
2. 0.5 fluid ounces of apple cider vinegar
3. 1 fluid ounce of coconut water
4. 1 cup of fragrance leaf

5. 0.5 ounce of olive oil and combined and boiling

DOSAGE

Take one shot after each meal for two months.

GALL BLADDER AND KIDNEY STONES REMOVER

Gallstones, also known as Cholelithiasis, are head deposits that form within the gall bladder, a tiny organ found below the liver on the right side of the belly. Gallstones can range in size from being smaller than a sand grain to being larger than a golf ball.

THE CAUSES

Pregnancy, obesity, diabetes, liver illness, a sedentary lifestyle, a high-fat diet, and some types of anemia are risk factors for gallstones. Individuals over the age of 60, women, and those of American Indian or Hispanic origin are more likely to have gallstones.

THE INDICATIONS

Many individuals get gallstones without being aware of it. Yet, when calculus blocks the bile duct. Symptoms include rapid onset of strong abdominal discomfort, especially on the right side, backache, nausea or vomiting, bloating, chills, and clay-colored feces. The duration of gallstone-related pain might range from minutes to hours.

NATURAL TREATMENTS

Gallstones can be quite painful and must be treated quickly. Consult your doctor for an accurate diagnosis and treatment. You can also employ a number of natural therapies to prevent and treat gallstones:

1. Over the first five days, drink four glasses of apple juice daily or consume four to five apples. Over these five days, when apple juice dissolves the gallstones, you should eat properly.

2. On the sixth day, refrain from eating dinner.

3. Take a teaspoon of Epsom salt (magnesium sulfate) with a glass of warm water about 6:00 p.m.

4. At 8:00 pm, repeat the process

5. At 10:00 p.m., combine a half-cup of olive oil with a half-cup of freshly squeezed lemon juice. Mix carefully and drink. The oil lubricates the stones and makes their passage easier. The following morning, you will discover green stones in the feces. Typically, there are 40-50 or even 100 stones on the floor; you may like to count them. Even if you have no symptoms of gallstones, it is always a good idea to cleanse the gallbladder with this natural treatment.

CURE TO GALLSTONE

1. VINEGAR FROM APPLES

The high acidity of vinegar from apples stops the liver from producing the most common form of gallstone-causing cholesterol. It also aids in the dissolution of gallstones and relieves discomfort. Drink on an empty stomach in the morning a blend of 2 spoon of vinegar from apples and 1 teaspoon of lemon liquid dissolved in a glass of warm water. Regular practice for two weeks can eliminate gallstones and alleviate pain.

2. LEMON

The formation of cholesterol is halted by lemon juice, which leads to a quicker recovery from gallstone strains. Pectin in lemon juice is believed to alleviate gallbladder pain caused by gallstones. Moreover, the vitamin C in lemon juice makes cholesterol more soluble in water, which expedites waste removal. Consume the juice of two freshly squeezed lemons in a glass of warm, fasting water every morning on an empty stomach, and continue this treatment for a week or longer if necessary.

3. CARROTS

When afflicted with cholelithiasis, it is vital to reduce fried and fatty foods for a week or two and follow a fruit and vegetable-based diet. A mixture of beetroot, cucumber, and carrot juice is an effective cure for gallstones. The beetroot cleanses the liver and fortifies the gallbladder. Cucumber's high water content is excellent for cleansing the liver and gallbladder. Carrots can be abundant in Vitamin C and other immune-boosting elements. Extract the juice from a cucumber and four medium-sized carrots. Combine them and consume this juice twice. Following this treatment for two weeks will result in a significant improvement in your condition.

PREPARATION

Every morning, there is one thing you should never fail to do. Warm honey water. Take a half glass of warm water and add two teaspoons of honey since it helps to cleanse the kidney, strengthen the heart, and enhance the immune system.

HEALTH TIPS / LIFESTYLE TO MAINTAIN YOUR KIDNEYS

Using paracetamol to prepare meat is the most efficient method for many households and restaurants; it saves gas, kerosene, or firewood and is significantly less expensive. One Sachet of 12 pills may be purchased for a small sum, and each tablet will soften a potful of meat in a matter of minutes; it appears to be a remarkable finding. But what they don't realize is that as much as they are shortening the cooking time, they are also shortening their time on mother earth. When eaten consistently (abuse), paracetamol is used to treat headaches and pains, but when boiled in a pot, it is a guaranteed express route to kidney or liver failure. Medical professionals specify when paracetamol may be used in cooking. It loses its analgesic properties and becomes extremely acidic and toxic for human consumption. As the method works, paracetamol is converted into 4-aminophenmol, which is particularly harmful to the kidneys and liver, according to doctors. In recent years, there has been an increase in the number of young men diagnosed with kidney failure, the majority of whom die as a result of substandard medical care. It is believed that consumption of paracetamol, Panadol, pepper soup, and the meat it is commonly used to prepare are contributing factors. Ignorance is expensive in this aspect. The Nigeria association of morphology (NAM) has also asserted that 25 million Nigerians, or over 13 percent of the country's estimated 180 million populations, suffer from chronic kidney disease. Yet, whereas paracetamol or Panadol are only harmful when heated, an overdose from daily use can still be fatal. FDA decreased the maximum dose of paracetamol (known as acetaminophen in the United States) in tablets and capsules to 325 mg in order to lessen the risk of accidental overdose. So, the recommendation is to take less paracetamol and pay attention to how your meat is prepared.

VITAL HEALTH INSTRUCTIONS

1. Respond to cellular phones using the left ear.

2. Do not combine your medication with cold water.

3. Do not consume a substantial meal after 5pm

4. Consume more water in the morning and less in the evening

5. The best time to sleep is between 10 p.m. and 4 a.m.

6. Do not lie down immediately after taking medication or eating.

7. Do not answer the phone while the battery is below one bar, as the radiation is 1,000 times stronger.

8. The underlying cause of the kidney disease epidemic in West Africa is monosodium glutamate (MSG), also known as "white Maggi."

It is present in magic sauce, magic cubes, Indomie, knor cubes, doyen cubes, and other flavor enhancers.

MSG is toxic to the kidney's glomerulus, which function as filters. Injury causes the kidneys to begin failing. Worse still, a feedback mechanism kicks in to help increase kidney function, but this results in hypertension, which leads to severe complications such as heart attack, stroke, and brain bleeding. You do not need MSG to enhance the flavor of your food in any way.

9. Use an abundance of onions with a small amount of table salt, dawadawa, lucus beans, turmeric, cinnamon, bay leaf, etc.

10. Consume ample amounts of water daily. It helps to dilute other toxic elements in meals and improves renal function.

11. Another killer is the sweetness or sugar substitutes found in the majority of frozen carbonated beverages.

Please use dates, honey, molasses, and cane sugar in place of sugar.

NUTRITIONALLY DENSE FOODS FOR INDIVIDUALS WITH KIDNEY AILMENT

Experts are identifying a growing number of links between chronic diseases, inflammation, and "supper food" that may prevent or protect against undesirable fatty acid oxidation, which occurs when oxygen in the system interacts with fats in the tissues and blood. Oxidation is an usual procedure of power generation and several chemical processes in the body, but uncontrolled reduction of fat and cholesterol generates molecules called free radicals that can harm your proteins, cellular membranes, and DNA.

Cardiovascular disease, cancer, Vascular dementia, Parkinson's disease, and other chronic and degenerative illnesses have been related to oxidative damage. Notwithstanding, phytonutrients foods can assist in eliminating free radicals and protecting the body. Many anti-oxidative foods are included in the kidney diet and are ideal alternatives for dialysis patients and those with chronic kidney disease (CKD). Because they experience increased inflammation and have a higher risk for cardiovascular disease, people with kidney disease must undertake certain lifestyle modifications, such as eating nutritious foods and working with a renal dietician to create a renal diet consisting of kidney-friendly foods.

1. RED BELL PEPPERS

- 1/4 cup red bell pepper
- 1mg salt 38mg potassium

Although red bell peppers are low in potassium and great in flavor, that is not the only reason they are perfect. These delicious vegetables are a wonderful source of vitamin A, vitamin B6, folic acid, and fiber for the kidney diet. Red bell peppers are beneficial because they contain lycopene, a cancer-fighting antioxidant. Use raw red bell peppers as an appetizer or snack, or include them into tuna or chicken salad. You may also roast peppers and use them as a topping for sandwiches or lettuce salads, cut them for an omelet, add them to grilled kabobs, or stuff them with ground turkey or beef and bake them for a man dish.

2. CABBAGE

- 12 cup of green cabbage
- 6mg sochum
- 10mg potassium
- 9mg phosphorus

As a cruciferous vegetable, cabbage is loaded with phytochemicals, which are chemical substances found in fruits and vegetables that neutralize free radicals. Many phytochemicals are also recognized to prevent and combat cancer and promote cardiovascular health. In addition to being rich in vitamin K, vitamin C, and fiber, cabbage is an inexpensive source of vitamin B6 and folic acid. It is an inexpensive supplement to the kidney diet. As slaw or a topping for fish tacos, raw cabbage is an excellent complement to a dialysis diet. It can be steamed, microwaved, or boiled and served with butter, cream cheese, pepper, or caraway seeds. If you are feeling sophisticated, shred cabbage with ground beef and bake it for a savory, nutrient-dense supper.

3. CAULIFLOWER

- 1/2 cup, boiling serving Cauliflower
- 9mg sodium 38mg potassium
- 20mg phosphorus

Cauliflower, another cruciferous vegetable, is rich in vitamin C and a strong source of folate and fiber. It is also loaded with indoles, glucosinolates, and thiocynates, which assist the liver in neutralizing harmful substances that could damage cell membranes and DNA. Serve it raw as crudités with a dipping sauce, incorporate it into a salad, steam or boil it, and season it with spices such as turmeric, curry powder, pepper, and herb seasoning. Also, you can prepare a non-dairy sauce, pour it over the cauliflower, and bake until cooked. You can mix cauliflower with paste or even mash cauliflower as a substitute for mashed potatoes on a dialysis diet.

4. GARLIC

- 1 bulb of garlic
- 1 mg sodium 12mg potassium
- 1mg phosphorus

Garlic prevents the formation of dental plaque, decreases cholesterol, and reduces inflammation. Add it to your meat after purchasing it fresh, bottled, minced, or powdered. Pasta or vegetable meals. Also, you can roast a head of garlic and spread it on bread. Garlic imparts a delectable flavor, and garlic powder is an excellent replacement for garlic salt in the dialysis diet.

5. ONIONS

- 1/2 cup portion of onion
- 8 mg sodium
- 116 mg potassium
- 8 mg phosphorus

Onion, a member of the allium family and a common ingredient in many recipes, contains sulfur compounds that contribute to its pungent odor. Yet, in addition to causing some individuals to shed tears. Onions are also abundant in flavonoids, including quercetin, a potent antioxidant that helps prevent heart disease and a variety of malignancies. Onions are low in potassium and rich in chromium, a mineral that aids in the metabolism of carbohydrates, fats, and proteins. Try using white, brown, and red onions, among others. Use raw onions on burgers, sandwiches, and salads, cook them and use them as a caramelized topping, or fry them into onion rings, and include onions in dishes such as Italian beef with peppers and onions.

6. APPLES

- 1 medium apple with peel
- 158mg sodium
- 10mg potassium,
- 10mg phosphorus.

Apples are known to lower cholesterol levels, decrease constipation, protect against cardiovascular disease, and reduce the rate of cancer. A daily apple, rich in fiber and anti-inflammatory chemicals, may keep the doctor away. Apples can be eaten raw, baked, made into apple sauce, or consumed as apple juice or apple cider in order to create a unique apple onion omelet.

7. CRANBERRIES

- 1/2 ounce of dried cranberries
- Juice cocktail
- 3mg sodium 22mg potassium
- 8mg phosphorus

- 14 cup of cranberry sauce contains 35 mg sodium
- 17 mg potassium
- 6 mg phosphorus.
- 1/2 ounce of dried cranberries

By preventing bacteria from adhering to the bladder wall, these tart, delectable berries are believed to protect against bladder infections. Similarly, cranberries protect the stomach against germs that cause ulcers and the lining of the gastrointestinal (GI) tract, so boosting GI health. Also, there is evidence that cranberries protect against cancer and heart disease. Cranberry items that are consumed most frequently are cranberry juice and cranberry sauce. Cranberries can also be added to salads or eaten as a snack.

8. BLUE BERRIES

- 1/2 cup serving of fresh blueberries
- 4 mg of sodium
- 35 mg of potassium
- 7 mg of phosphorus.

Blueberries are rich in anti-inflammatory phytonutrients known as anthocyanidins, which give them their blue color, and are packed with antioxidant phytonutrients. Blueberries are an excellent source of vitamin C, manganese, a chemical that promotes healthy bones, and filtering agents. They may also aid in protecting the brain against the causes of aging. Antioxidants in blueberries and other berries have been found to reduce bone resorption in estrogen-deficient mice. Purchase fresh, frozen, or dried blueberries and use them in cereal or fruit smoothies with whipped topping. Also available is blueberry juice.

1. **RASPBERRIES**

- 1/2 cup portion of raspberries
- 10 mg sodium
- 93 mg potassium
- 7 mg phosphorus

Raspberries include ellagic acid, a phytonutrient that neutralizes free radicals in the body to prevent cell damage. They also include flavonoids known as anthocycinins, which are antioxidants responsible for their red color. Raspberries, a great source of manganese, vitamin C, fiber, and folate, a B vitamin, may have qualities that hinder the growth and creation of cancer cells. Add raspberries to cereal, puree and sweeten them to create a dessert sauce, or include them into vinaigrette.

10. STRAWBERRIES

- 1/2 cup strawberries
- 1mg sodium
- 120mg potassium
- 13mg phosphorus

Strawberries are abundant in the phenolic compounds, anthocyanins and ellagitannins.

ANTHOCYANINS: which give strawberries their red hue, are potent antioxidants that aid in the protection of cell structures and the prevention of oxidative damage. Strawberries are an outstanding source of vitamin C, manganese, and fiber. They are recognized for their heart-protecting, anti-cancer, and anti-inflammatory properties. Strawberries can be consumed with cereal smoothies and salad, sliced and served fresh, or topped with whipped topping. If you want a more sophisticated dessert, you can sweeten strawberry pudding, sorbet, or puree to serve as a dessert.

11. CHERRIES

- 1/2 ounce of fresh cherries
- 10mg sodium
- 160mg potassium
- 15mg phosphorous

Daily consumption of cherries has been demonstrated to lessen inflammation. They are also loaded with heart-protecting antioxidants and polyphenols. Consume fresh cherries as a snack or prepare a cherry sauce to accompany hog or lamb. This delicious dish can also be consumed in the form of cherry juice.

12. RED GRAPES

- 1ounce portion of red grapes
- 1mg sodium
- 38mg potassium
- 4mg phosphorus

The reddish hue of red grapes is due to the presence of flavonoids. Flavonoids protect against heart disease by preventing oxidation and lowering the formation of blood clots. Resveratrol, a flavonoid found in grapes, may also enhance the generation of nitric oxide, which relaxes blood vessel muscle cells to improve blood flow. Moreover, these flavonoids protect against cancer and reduce inflammation.

Buy grapes with red or purple skin, as they contain more anthocyanin, and freeze them for a snack or to quench the thirst of individuals on a fluid restriction diet for dialysis. Add grapes to a chicken salad or fruit salad. Use grapes in a creative kidney diet recipe for turkey kabods. They can also be consumed as grape juice.

13. EGG WHITES

- 2 beaten egg whites
- 7 grams' protein
- 110mg sodium
- 108mg phosphorus

Egg whites are pure protein and provide the finest quality protein with all the essential amino acids for the kidney diet. Moreover, egg whites have less phosphorus than other protein sources, such as egg yolk or meats. By using fresh, powdered, or pasteurized egg whites. Create an omelet or egg white sandwich, or include pasteurized egg whites into smoothies or drinks. To increase protein, create egg snacks or add egg whites or hard-boiled eggs to a salad.

14. OLIVE OIL

- 1 tablespoon olive oil
- 10mg phosphorus

Olive oil is an excellent source of anti-inflammatory oleic acid. Olive oil's monounsaturated content protects against oxidation. Olive oil is abundant in anti-inflammatory and antioxidant polyphenols and phytochemicals. According to studies, populations that use a lot of olive oil as opposed to other oils had reduced rates of heart disease and cancer. Get virgin or extra-virgin olive oil, as they contain more antioxidants. Use olive oil for salad dressing, cooking, bread dipping, and vegetable marinating.